A Doctor's Basic Business Handbook

To Jay —
Thanks again for visiting
us down in Georgia, and for
carrying our golf team! You'll always
be "BIG PLAY JAY" to us! Cheers!

Brad

*Practical Strategies for Success
in the Real World of Medicine*

A DOCTOR'S
BASIC BUSINESS
HANDBOOK

*Things I Wish I Had Known
When I Got Started*

Brandon D. Bushnell, MD, MBA

*Team Bushnell Publishing
Rome, GA, USA*

A Doctor's Basic Business Handbook:
Things I Wish I Had Known When I Got Started
Copyright 2015 by Brandon D. Bushnell
First edition

ISBN-13:978-0692493571

ISBN-10:0692493573

Library of Congress Control Number: 2015916778

Publisher: Team Bushnell Publishing, Rome, GA, USA

Book design by Alan Pranke

PRINTED IN THE UNITED STATES OF AMERICA

Dedication:

To the amazing teachers I've been blessed to have in my life who taught me how to write: Shirley Marks, Marcia Davis, George Harwood, Vereen Bell, and – most of all – my mom, Betsy Bushnell.

And To Pop – Who taught me that in medicine, caring and character are everything.

Praise for

THINGS I WISH I HAD KNOWN

This book serves as an excellent reference to learn about the world beyond formal medical education. Dr. Bushnell explains several key topics in a very practical and readable concise format. I will definitely recommend it to all of my medical students, residents, fellows, and early career colleagues.

—Hassan R. Mir, MD, MBA, FACS
Director of Orthopaedic Residency Program, University of South Florida
Director of Trauma Research, Florida Orthopaedic Institute, Tampa, FL

I can't really summarize all the mistakes I've made and naiveté I've displayed over the years in encountering the issues Dr Bushnell brings up in this timely book. Perhaps a little more concentration on the nuts and bolts of a practice and not just orthopedic learning would have been very beneficial for me. Dr Bushnell summarizes many things I truly "wish I had known" and I would strongly recommend you take advantage of this information and save a few costly missteps.

—Robert T. Burks, MD
Professor, Orthopedic Surgery
Director, Sports Medicine Fellowship
University of Utah, Salt Lake City, UT

Dr. Bushnell's book is a "must-read" for every new physician (and many who have been in practice)! He clearly explains many of the issues associated with the business of medicine that we were never taught in medical school.

—Douglas W. Lundy, MD, MBA, FACS
co-President, Resurgens Orthopaedics
Atlanta, Georgia

This little book is a gem, particularly for newer physicians. Dr. Bushnell offers a straightforward checklist of key issues to consider and pithy and wise advice about effectively managing one's life and practice. I think most physicians will find multiple nuggets of insight from this quick read.

—**Stanley Harris, Ph.D.**
Former Academic Director, Physicians Executive MBA Program
Associate Dean, Graduate & International Programs
Torchmark Professor
Harbert College of Business, Auburn University, Auburn, AL

Dr. Bushnell has leveraged his expertise and insights into a timely and much needed publication: *A Doctor's Basic Business Handbook.* Yes there are many things I wish I had known before I started my career as an orthopedic surgeon! This publication addresses those gaps in recognizing and addressing strategies for entering clinical practice and realizing success. It here-and-now as far as dealing with our rapidly evolving healthcare system, as well as comprehensive and practical. As I currently chair an orthopedic department that includes 47 residents and 120 attendings, I believe this book is a must-read for all orthopedists in training as well as faculty.

—**Nicholas A. Sgaglione, M.D.**
Professor and Chair
Department of Orthopaedic Surgery
Hofstra North Shore – Long Island Jewish School of Medicine
Senior Vice President & Executive Director
North Shore – Long Island Jewish Health System
Great Neck, NY

Medical school rarely prepares physicians for the significant business decisions that have a major impact on their happiness, income, and quality of life. A few hours reading Dr. Bushnell's book will provide value throughout a physician's career.

—**David M. Glaser, J.D.**
Fredrikson & Byron Law Firm
Minneapolis, MN

Dr. Bushnell's book is a superb resource for young physicians, particularly those facing contract negotiations as they start independent practice after training.

—**Peter G. Robertson, M.D.**
Cardiac Electrophysiology
Saint Thomas Heart
Murfreesboro, TN

A Doctor's Basic Business Handbook should be at the top of the list for every senior resident and young physician in practice. Dr. Bushnell summarizes the most important issues and breaks them down into understandable terms. This valuable resource will provide clear direction in the otherwise murky waters of contracts, healthcare law, and other issues facing physicians.

—**John C. Browning, MD, FAAD, FAAP**
Texas Dermatology and Laser Specialists
Chief of Dermatology
Children's Hospital of San Antonio
Assistant Professor, Baylor College of Medicine
San Antonio, TX

While medical schools and residency programs do a fantastic job training physicians to practice medicine, virtually none teach anything about health care or personal economics. This book helps to fill a part of that void.

—**Thomas William Baker, J.D.**
Baker Donelson Law Firm
Atlanta, GA

This handbook is perfect for the young doctor in training and or those starting practice. In fact it would even be very helpful for those of us who have been in practice for a number of years. It is organized, clear and concise and gets to the point of what we need to know about the financial implications of practice. We are grateful to Dr. Bushnell for sharing this handbook with us. It can only make us more aware of the aspects of medicine that are lacking in our training.

—**Richard Hawkins, MD**
Fellowship Director, Steadman Hawkins Sports Medicine Program
Professor of Surgery, University of South Carolina
Adjunct Professor, Clemson University
Greenville, SC

Dr. Bushnell provides sound advice for the early-career physician, offering tangible ways to achieve personal and professional success in an era of rapidly-evolving health care delivery. I recommend his book to anyone looking to avoid many of the mistakes and pitfalls that befall so many well-intentioned young doctors."

—**J. Kyle Horton, MD**
Endocrinologist, Greenville Health System
Clinical Assistant Professor, University of South Carolina School of
Medicine- Greenville, SC

Given my personal background in the business world of IT and finance with medicine as a second career, I've consistently witnessed colleagues looking for guidance into the business side of medicine. Exposure to real world financial fundamentals during medical school and residency is essentially absent, and the average physician is unprepared to make educated financial decisions. Dr. Bushnell's book is a must-have for all doctors and students to help navigate through pitfalls of business while focusing on patient care.

—**Patrick C. Kindregan, D.O.**
Chief Resident – Family Medicine
Floyd Medical Center
Rome, GA

Dr. Bushnell hits a home run with this comprehensive, easily understood business manual for the practice of medicine. He covers all of the topics we really need to know but are rarely taught during our training.

—**Thomas Noonan, MD**
Head Team Physician, Colorado Rockies
Steadman Hawkins Clinic Denver
Denver, CO

I highly recommend this book to anyone stepping into the medical world. Dr. Bushnell has authored a thorough guide that delves into the business side of medicine; an anthology of medical business teaching that only comes with experience. You have gone through school and have the medical training you need to succeed, in this book are the specific tools that will enable you to take your practice to the next level and flourish in the business world of medicine that we live in.

—**Misty Suri, M.D.**
Team Physician, New Orleans Saints
Team Physician, New Orleans Pelicans
Sports Medicine and Orthopaedic Surgery
Ochsner Health System
New Orleans, LA

TABLE OF CONTENTS

Introduction 1

Ch 1: Ten Points You Need to Know About Contracts 3

Ch 2: Top Ten Points of Effectively Managing Your Personal Finances 15

Ch 3: Make-Or Break Basics of Industry and Hospital Relationships 27

Ch 4: Tips from the Trenches on Billing, Coding, and Pricing 43

Ch 5: How "To Be" Successful in Marketing Your Practice 55

Final Thoughts 67

Additional Resources. 69

About the Author 71

Introduction

The business world of health care is fascinating, in no small part because it is unlike any other sector of the American economy. Although it is one of the largest dollar-amount components of our gross national product, health care does not play by any of the business rules that typically apply to everything else. Indeed, my wife, a CPA who previously worked in health care finance at a prominent health care system, would often ask her bosses, "Why is this so different? The way we manage this makes no sense!" and their reply was usually, "Well, that's just health care."

As a pre-med major in college, a medical student, a resident, a fellow, and an early-career physician or surgeon, you probably have not had a lot of formal exposure to the "dark side" of health care—the *business side*. We spend most of our time learning clinical things like current controversies in colorectal surgery, the interactions of statins with anti-psychotics, or the best choice of graft type for ACL reconstruction. Unfortunately, we have likewise wasted a lot of time on practically irrelevant trivia like the steps of the Krebs cycle and the role of the Christmas Factor in the clotting cascade.

Unless you had the foresight to take a business class or two along the way, or had the time to read about contract law between skimming the latest edition of the *New England Journal of Medicine*, you are probably like most other doctors in training or in the early stages of practice. You are armed to the teeth with medical knowledge, but completely defenseless when it comes to understanding business issues.

I took my first "business" class (*Introduction to Accounting*) as a senior at Vanderbilt for the sole purpose of being able to "talk accounting" with my then-girlfriend, now-wife. However, not long after I had entered the "real world" of private practice several years ago, I realized I should have paid *much closer attention*. I was confronted with terms like "restrictive covenants," "accrual accounting," "Stark Law implications," and "CPT versus MS-DRG valuation of service." I realized I was adrift in a strange new sea where my ability to stay afloat depended not only on how quickly I could resect a meniscus, but also on how well I could interpret a spreadsheet.

Over my first few years in practice, my large, multi-specialty group hosted several seminars designed to teach us more about the business of medicine, and I became drawn to learn more. I decided to go back to school and earn a degree at Auburn University's Physician Executive MBA program—a truly enlightening experience. As a recent graduate, by no means do I pretend to be an expert in all matters of the business of health care, but I certainly know *a whole lot more* than I did straight out of my sports medicine fellowship.

With these experiences in mind, I developed this book as part of the curriculum for the 2015 Metcalf Winter Meeting of the Arthroscopy Association of North America. It is designed to help those of you with a similar need for or interest in some of the *"things I wish I had known when I got started."* I hope you will find the topics and information to be both engaging and valuable.

—Brandon D. Bushnell, MD, MBA

Chapter 1

TEN POINTS YOU NEED TO
KNOW ABOUT CONTRACTS

Even before the signing of the Magna Carta in 1215 A.D., contracts have formed the backbone of Western civilization. The business world today runs on contracts, and a basic understanding of them is essential to any early-career doctor. Contract issues can make or break your happiness. Hopefully you would not get married on a whim, and you should approach your contract with a similar level of serious review and deliberation. While you might think you have found the "perfect job," a bad contract can ruin even the most ideal situation. Ultimately, you should have *every* contract reviewed by an experienced legal professional.

I have compiled a list of the "Top Ten Points" of contracts as a basic framework for understanding these important documents, with much credit given to Tom Baker, Esq., my law professor at Auburn, for helping to put it into understandable terms for doctors. He has a wonderful medical law book that I highly recommend (the latest edition is pending publication).

1. Enforceability (Verbal vs. Written)

Ultimately the power of an agreement between two parties matters, but *only if* the parties under the agreement can be forced to do what they agree to do. The legal distinction between a promise (which people make every day, often to break later) and a contract is the *enforceability* of the contract. At its heart, a contract is nothing more than an enforceable promise.

Three legal elements comprise an enforceable promise: an offer, an acceptance, and consideration (see below). Offer and acceptance, taken together, make up the concept of "mutual assent" or a "meeting of the minds."

Depending on state law, verbal contracts often have legal enforceability if the components of mutual assent and consideration have transpired. As you negotiate with potential employers or groups in any setting – not just for a job, but for other business deals as well – watch what you say, as a statement and a handshake might land you in an *assumed verbal contract*. For example, saying to a managing partner, "I'm looking forward to working for your group, and making $500K a year," can result in that partner holding you responsible for actually joining the group, since offer, acceptance, and consideration have transpired. Ultimately, the wise saying, "get it in writing," is always the best policy to follow. You might not completely understand an agreement unless it is written down, which allows you to review it as many times as needed. A written version also enables friends and advisors to review it. In some states, agreements involving dollar amounts above a certain number may be *required* to be in written form.

Don't be afraid to go through multiple drafts of a document before you sign it, as your signature confirms that you recognize and agree that all three legal elements (an offer, an acceptance, and consideration) exist, thus sealing the enforceability of that document. If a contract might be grossly unfair, it does *not* mean it is not enforceable—a time-honored concept known as "folly is not fraud." This means that you cannot claim exemption from the provisions of a contract *because* it is a bad deal for you, or that you "didn't know any better."

You will be bound to the contract, even if it results in events that hurt your finances or your career. If you sign a bad contract, you are stuck.

2. Consideration

The term *consideration* refers to something of value that is given in exchange for a promise. This is a key, critical concept that distinguishes an enforceable promise (i.e., a contract) from an unenforceable promise. Under a contract, each side usually provides something of value, or consideration, to the other. Consideration could take the form of money, services provided, hard assets, intellectual property, and many other things that one side can provide to the other. In the example of an employment contract, the doctor provides the consideration of his or her professional services in exchange for the consideration of a salary from the hospital.

Pay close attention to the language governing "consideration," as it should clearly state *what each side will receive from the other.*

3. Compensation and Benefit Structure

From your perspective, *consideration* could be the primary key to the contract. As you come out of training and start your career, one of your most pressing questions will probably be, "How much am I going to get paid?" The answers might seem simple: "$500K per year for two years," or "$30K a month." Contractual structure of compensation and benefits, however, can be much more complicated than it may initially appear.

Because compensation and benefits constitute "consideration," their presence makes the contract enforceable.

Compensation structure can take on countless forms. Most contracts involve some sort of fixed salary, as very few employers would expect a new physician to accept an "eat-what-you-kill" structure directly out of training. (*Note – "eat-what-you-kill" is a term commonly used in reference to a purely*

5

production-based salary. That is, you "eat," or enjoy reimbursement directly related to what you "kill," or the revenue you generate.) Indeed, it usually takes several months or years for you to build up sufficient volume to generate enough revenue to cover your expenses. In recognition of this process of establishing a practice, many contracts involve a salary guarantee for a fixed period of time, with the employer assuming the loss if expenses are not covered – and enjoying the gain if you happen to generate more revenue than expense. Some contracts include provisions for bonus payments if your revenue exceeds expenses; such bonuses are offered as a means of incentivizing you to work harder and to reach higher volume numbers. Calculations can be based on Relative Value Units (RVU's–see **Chapter 4**), dollars billed, dollars collected, or other such measures of performance. Be sure that you understand the method used in your situation and that this method is delineated very clearly in the contract and/or a direct supporting document (such as your employer's operating agreement or bylaws).

Perhaps the most important aspect of analyzing your compensation structure—and one that usually does not always appear in the contract directly—is making sure that your workload matches your compensation. Employers are unlikely to pay you at the 95th percentile of first-year salaries if you do only 50 cases per year or see only 3 patients per day; but employers will be more than happy to pay you in the 5th percentile of first-year salaries if you perform 700 annual surgeries, see 75 patients daily in the office, and generate ridiculous levels of revenue on their behalf. You can use data from the Medical Group Management Association (MGMA) or other similar entities to help determine relative levels of compensation and workload.

**Be sure you get paid fairly for the level of work
that you will be expected to do.**

A "hidden" feature of the compensation structure is the "benefits package" or "benefit structure" of the contract. Sometimes these items are included in the actual contract, but more frequently they appear in a supporting document (such as an employee manual, bylaws, or operating agreement). Benefits packages can be widely variable, but should generally include:

1. Health insurance–this should also include options for coverage for dependents.

2. Disability insurance–a critical feature for a surgeon or other proceduralist.

3. Retirement investment options–such as a 401k or 403b plan.

4. Life insurance–included less frequently than the first three benefits above.

5. Extras.

"Extras" can be everything from discounted laundry and dry cleaning services to country club or civic group memberships. Many contracts involve stipulations for extra funding for Continuing Medical Education (CME) or "professional development." Try to get your Board exam fees, society memberships, and other professional expenses included as well. First-time contracts might offer loan repayment offers, moving allowances, or other features designed to entice you to take a job. Some private practices might set up "company car" arrangements for partners, which is a nice feature if you are driving to satellite offices or outreach clinics.

Be sure that you calculate the *true value*
of the benefit structure as you negotiate your contract,
and that the benefits are clearly stated in writing.

4. Term and Termination

Two of the simplest and most important aspects of a contract are 1) "how long does it last?" (*Term*), and 2) "how do the parties get out of it?" (*Termination*). The term of a contract is usually expressed in months or years. Many contracts have an "evergreen" clause, which provides for automatic renewal year-to-year, but others have a fixed expiration date with no provision for renewal.

**Do *not* assume that your contract has
an evergreen clause—be sure to confirm it.**

As long as both parties are happy under a contract, termination will not be an issue. However, if either party seeks to end the contractual relationship, the provisions of the termination clause become absolutely critical. Central to termination is the concept of *cause*, or the reason for termination. Most contracts have a "without cause" provision, which gives a set time period of advance notice after which either party can end the relationship for any reason. More importantly, each side usually has a list of reasons for which they can end the contract immediately or on very short notice—that is, "with cause." For example, an employer may have "cause" to terminate the contract if the employee is convicted of a felony; likewise, the employee could have "cause" to terminate the contract if the employer files for bankruptcy.

**The term and termination clauses of a contract can literally dictate
the course of your professional life. They should be analyzed
with extreme scrutiny.**

5. Breach and Remedy

The concept of *breach* seems simple at first – a breach is one party's failure to fulfill its contractual obligations. A doctor's complete failure to show up for work, for example, would be a breach of an employment contract. Depending on the specific wording of a contract, however, something as innocuous as her late dictation of charts could also be construed as a breach. Most contracts have clear definitions of what constitutes a breach of the agreement and of how one side notifies the other side of this breach. Beware of references to secondary documents, such as operating agreements, bylaws, or other lists of "rules" that can introduce a long list of potential contractual breaches, and therefore entail more risk exposure for you.

The contract should have provisions for *remedy* – or how to repair a breach. Hopefully, each side will still want to maintain their contractual relationship and work through the breach. Remedy clauses should cover the communication process between the parties, provide a timeframe under which the breach should be resolved, and – most importantly – a description of what happens if the breach is *not* resolved. Usually, an unresolved breach becomes a reason for termination of the contract.

Remedy clauses should not place an excessive burden on you, and should likewise give you appropriate power to recover potential losses caused by a breach by the other party. For example, in most situations, an employer should not be able to both *fire* you and then also *fine* you on the way out. Furthermore, you should have the ability to recover financial compensation if the employer does not provide the agreed-upon office space or appropriate support staff as stated in an employment contract.

6. Restrictive Covenants (AKA Non-Compete Clauses)

One of the most emotional and powerful aspects of many medical contracts is the *restrictive covenant*—or the dreaded "non-compete clause." In general, this clause specifically prohibits the employee from providing services that compete with the former employer within both a specific time period and a specific geographic region. Non-compete clauses and their legality differ by state. In general, however, the "reasonableness" test governs the enforceability of these clauses. The provisions must be deemed "reasonable" in terms of time, territory, and activity. For example, if the clause prohibits "the practice of arthroscopic surgery within a twenty-mile radius of the employer for one year," then it is probably reasonable. If it prohibits "any practice of medicine in the continental United States for twenty years," then it is probably not. Finally, most of these clauses have some sort of penalty associated with the violation of them—such as you paying one year's worth of salary to your former employer if you stay in town and join a rival employer.

**Be sure you understand the specifics of any non-compete clause.
If *it is* reasonable, then you will likely be held responsible
for any penalties associated with it.**

More importantly, restrictive covenants can include non-solicitation, confidentiality, and non-disparagement clauses. This "fine print" covers prohibitions against 1) recruiting patients or staff from your former employer to join you at your new employer, 2) transferring medical records, and 3) holding onto other intellectual property. They might even prohibit you from saying bad things in public about your former employer. These clauses can prove as onerous as the traditional geographic- and time-specific restrictions.

7. Stark Laws/Kickback Implications

Together, a group of federal laws known as the "Stark Laws," and the federal Anti-Kickback Statute, govern almost every situation in health care in which money changes hands (See Chapter 3 for more details). Obviously, this includes contracts involving physicians. Things that might be perfectly legal, and sometimes commonplace, in contracts in other industries (such as real estate), could represent a major violation of one of these federal laws in health care. While a detailed discussion of these laws is far beyond the scope of this document, *remember this take-home point:*

**Every contract you will ever sign as a physician will have
potential Stark Law and Anti-Kickback implications.
Be sure that you understand *exactly* what they are, and that
you are not in violation of these regulations. If you do not
completely understand them, do *not* sign the contract. In the modern
medical-legal environment, the specifics of these laws, their interpretation,
and their application are constantly changing. It is thus critical to seek
professional help from someone familiar with the latest updates.**

8. Ownership of Patients, Medical Records, and Intellectual Property

As discussed above, restrictive covenants in a contract may define who actually "owns" the *patients* of a physician's practice. You do not want to spend years building wonderful relationships with your patients only to then discover that you have been doing all of that work to create patients who are "locked into" the hospital that just fired you. A contract should specifically describe your rights to patient access after termination of the agreement. Even if you move far away, your contract could still affect your relationships with patients.

Likewise, a contract should describe who actually "owns" *medical records* created during the course of working under the contract. If you change employers, yet still retain many of your former patients, the transfer of records (or lack thereof) can be a *major* issue of transition. Sometimes, your patients could be forced to bear the actual cost of transferring records. Worse still, your former employer could potentially hit you with a major fee for transferring multiple patients' records at one time.

Both of these issues generally fall under state law, and thus they will differ by practice location. Be sure to have your contract reviewed by a lawyer familiar with the specific laws applicable to your particular geographic location and area of practice.

Another important "ownership" item is that of *intellectual property*. If you are taking an academic job, or maybe a partial academic position (i.e., private practice with academic appointment), this issue can be critical. Your employer can claim any form of intellectual property—such as writings, equipment designs, or business models—in its entirety or in part. In other words, your employer *may have rights* to whatever you invent, write, or otherwise create.

For example, let's imagine that in your job as an associate professor at a major university hospital, you invent a new type of suture anchor for arthroscopic rotator cuff repair or create a new algorithm for managing pediatric sepsis. Unless your intellectual property is protected in your contract, any royalties or other compensation that might arise from its eventual sale or marketing may actually go to the *hospital*, and you will receive absolutely nothing for your efforts.

Negotiate intellectual property protections into your contract if you can, although some large academic centers may not budge on this issue. Even in private practice, you want to be sure (if possible) that you can protect your intellectual property rights in the contract. Sometimes presentations or talks you give (see **Chapter 3**) can be considered intellectual property, so be sure you have this issue clearly spelled out in your contract.

9. Governing Law

As mentioned above, the laws that govern contracts vary by state. A short clause in most contracts is the "governing law" clause—which, simply, declares the state (and sometimes, the city) whose laws will govern the contract. While it might seem like a formality, this clause can mean the difference in who wins or loses if a dispute arises. Especially if you are moving to a new state (such as in a locum tenens situation, or changing jobs), this clause is critical. As above, make sure your lawyer and/or advisor understands the specific laws that will govern your contract.

10. Entire Agreement

The *entire agreement* clause, which is a seemingly "vanilla" clause that in fact has great hidden power, is generally veiled within the boring boilerplate provisions near the end of the document. In short, it provides that the contract constitutes the entire agreement between the two parties, and that all prior agreements, whether verbal or written, are now merged into the present document. This is critically important if you have an associate's contract and are now signing on as a partner, or if you had some sort of "recruitment agreement" prior to signing your actual employment contract. If there are differences between earlier contracts and the later one, then the later one supersedes under the entire agreement clause.

For example, let us suppose that you sign a contract as an associate that has a few nice clauses governing benefit structure, bonus compensation, and vacation days that all are in your favor. As part of the "carrot" designed to get you to come to town, your employer threw in these clauses so that you would have a $30,000 holiday bonus, a guaranteed six weeks of vacation, and fully paid health, dental, life, and disability insurance.

These clauses, however, are not included in your partnership-level employment contract, but the new contract does indeed have an *"entire agreement"* clause. By signing the new contract *without* the other clauses in it, you are essentially agreeing to leave them out. That means no benefits, no bonus, and no vacation. There is no automatic carry-forward, and the "entire agreement" clause wipes out the enforceability of any prior contract once the new one is signed.

Take-home point—when you sign a new contract with a party with whom you have previous agreements or contracts, make sure that the new contract contains *everything* from prior agreements that you want to have in it.

BONUS: Negotiations ... *Because it's so important*

Entire classes are taught about negotiations. Indeed, some people make careers out of negotiating (see Kevin Spacey and Samuel L. Jackson in *The Negotiator*). For our purposes, understand one thing: *everything is negotiable.* Depending on multiple factors, each side of a negotiation has something that the other side needs or wants. Each side will have relative strengths and weaknesses. If the other side in your negotiation has much more strength, you may not be able to get every single provision in the contract to go your way – but that doesn't mean you shouldn't try. Understand both your position and that of the other party, get professional advice, and then work to create the best possible contract for yourself, while at the same time respecting the other side in the process.

Many who advise about negotiations will emphasize various aspects of deals and contracts, with certain factors becoming more or less important on an individual basis. For example, if the location of a job is your top priority (such as in your hometown), then salary and benefits could be forced into a secondary role. However, almost all professional negotiators will agree upon the critical importance of the "Best Alternative to a Negotiated Agreement" (BATNA).

The BATNA is your proverbial "Plan B" option if things in the negotiation simply do not work out between you and the other party at the negotiating table. If you are negotiating an employment contract with a potential employer, then your BATNA might be a job with another employer in the same market or in another town. If negotiations are not going your way, and you know that your BATNA is perhaps a better deal than the one developing at hand, then you can confidently walk away from the negotiation. On the other hand, if you don't know what your other options could be, then you hold a much weaker position in the current negotiation.

A "Best Alternative to a Negotiated Agreement" (BATNA) illustrates that everything, including the negotiation process itself, *is negotiable.*

Chapter 2

TOP TEN POINTS OF EFFECTIVELY MANAGING YOUR PERSONAL FINANCES

While some early-career physicians and surgeons can find themselves in charge of their own practice, the solo practice and isolated small group practice models have become increasingly antiquated. For the brave souls who go into such situations, this book is far too basic for your needs. For most others, however, you can hopefully trust the leadership roles in the business of managing your practice to more experienced individuals as you "learn the ropes." Meanwhile, however, almost every single doctor will still likely be the captain of his or her own *personal* financial ship. As such, I have created a "Top Ten Points of Effectively Managing Your Personal Finances" to help you as you set out. Additionally, I would strongly recommend buying a wonderful book that I have found extremely helpful: *Doctor's Eyes Only: Exclusive Financial Strategies for Today's Doctors and Dentists* (see **Additional Resources**).

1. Don't "Act Rich"

Unlike most other careers, one of the most interesting things about the finances of physicians is that after residency, most doctors will "add a zero" to the right side of their annual paycheck. Being thrown into this situation of "sudden money" – with no business background and having lived very frugally for many years – can have dangerous implications on the personal level. Many doctors attempt to "act rich" by making big-ticket purchases such as a large home, a vacation home, a luxury car, or other such items, sometimes even before they have drawn their first paycheck. You will be flooded with offers of high levels of easy credit, "special loans," and other such financial traps, making it easier to *act as rich* as you want to be.

Stated plainly, "acting rich" will probably keep you from ever actually *being* rich. Live within your means, and you will likely have plenty of money for the "fun" stuff later.

One of the most common mistakes young physicians make is assuming that their first job position will be their last. In my field of orthopedics, recent statistics indicate that over half of all surgeons will change employers within the first two years after training. Many physicians will change multiple times. Unfortunately, many doctors decide to start "putting down roots" in their new town before they have adequately learned a whole lot about it. Sometimes the new place might not fit your tastes, it might be too far from family, or it simply might not be the place for you for any number of reasons. Roots are not bad in their own right, but they can create problems if you try to develop them too deeply too quickly.

For example, I started my practice in my current position within weeks of when an anesthesiologist colleague started her practice. She bought a home for around $700,000, but at our two-year mark, she discovered that her group had decided *not* to make her a partner. She was unable to find another job in town, or even in one of the nearby communities. She sold the home almost a year later (after she and her family had moved to another state)—for almost *half* of the purchase price. Now, she is still burdened by payments on a $350,000 loan on *someone else's house*. Had she rented or bought a less-expensive home during her "probationary" early period of practice, she would not be saddled with such a gigantic level of debt. Unfortunately, such "horror stories" are not uncommon with new doctors. Try not to be one of them.

If you are married, be sure that your spouse understands this same concept. Many a physician's spouse, who has "suffered" through the trying times of training, can feel that she or he is entitled to a larger house, a nice car, a country club membership, or other such luxuries as a "reward" for persevering through the leaner years. While this attitude may be justified in some respects, such a sense of entitlement can drive poor decision-making in the early days of your career.

This is not to say that you should not try to make your first job work out. No one likes a "vagabond doc" with a history of jumping ship multiple times. In fact, you could find it harder to get another job if you don't have a history of keeping one for a meaningful period of time. Nevertheless, you do need to respect the fact that things might not work out, in spite of your best intentions and efforts. Start by making decisions and purchases that do not "tie you down" too much and that preserve your ability to be mobile if you have to change situations. If things do work out, and as your finances improve, you can always upgrade.

Bad decisions or "downgrades" will haunt you and your family forever, whereas the rewards of celebrating with an appropriate upgrade can be some of the proudest moments of your life.

2. Build a Team

Like surgeons who need a team in the OR to manage even a simple case, you need a team to manage your personal financial matters. The key components to this team include:

1. Lawyer.

2. Accountant.

3. Financial Planner.

These individuals should be chosen for their wisdom, experience, and integrity. Particular experience with health care or physicians can be an added benefit. Beware picking teammates who are family members or pre-existing close friends, because a mix of personal and professional relationships can prove volatile or possibly catastrophic. If you are new to an area, do your homework. Acquire information from colleagues and friends, but also investigate your potential team members on your own using the Internet, the local Chamber of Commerce or Better Business Bureau, and other resources. In the digital age, don't rule out team members who are in business elsewhere geographically, especially if you already have had a well-established relationship with them. In many cases, having more than one of each team member could be beneficial, but you should have one person at each position that you consider your "primary" contact.

3. Manage Cash Flow

One of the most important concepts to comprehend in the early years of practice is that of cash flow. This issue can be summarized as:

**"You will *make* a lot of money, but you will not
have a lot of money."**

As you begin your practice, and establish a post-training lifestyle, bills will quickly add up as your spending habits inevitably rise to meet your new income level. It is critical to appropriately manage your actual *cash* and money in other forms that can be easily accessed and moved around (such as savings and checking accounts, money market accounts, etc.). For example, if the air conditioning unit on your new house breaks, but you don't have enough money in the bank to pay for the repairs, how will you get it fixed? Credit card? Loan from parents? While such options can work, they may have drawbacks, such as accrued interest and injured pride.

**Make a point to study, understand, and manage your
own personal cash flow.**

Perhaps the first and most important step you should take in managing cash flow is to establish an "emergency" or "rainy-day" fund. This should be a checking or money-market account or another readily available form of money that you can access quickly. This fund is not a "slush fund" for frivolous purchases or "fun stuff." Instead, it is a "safety net" of money to help you if you suddenly run into an unexpected major expense and/or suffer a sudden loss of income. The size of this fund can vary, but three to six months' worth of income is probably a good target. Additional savings are important, too, and we discuss that idea more under "investments."

Another important step is to minimize your use of *actual* cash. In today's digital world, very few transactions are completely and obligatorily cash-only. Using digital transactions can make them easier to trace, record, analyze, and manage. You will find budgeting and financial planning very difficult if you have no idea where your money actually goes every month. Many banks offer budgeting software and other such support for those who use their debit cards. Many people might use a credit card almost exclusively for their day-to-day expenditures, thus enjoying benefits such as travel or purchase discounts, reward points or "miles," the ability to dispute or cancel erroneous transactions, and added protections in cases of identity theft. Be sure, of course, to pay the card's balance every month if you use this approach. Don't let the card become "free money" that lands you in debt trouble.

4. Manage Risk

In medicine, we are taught from the early days of medical school (as well as in college) to *fear* medical-legal risk. But we get very little help in actually *understanding* it. Beyond the basics of "document everything," and "CYA," risk remains a scary and nebulous subject. In our personal lives, we have a similar lack of understanding, but perhaps we lack the fear that exists in our professional lives and motivates us to action. Unfortunately, there often is no concrete distinction between our personal and professional risks, as events in one area will always affect the other. You should therefore approach risk management from a *global* viewpoint. Understand any and every way in which the things you have worked so hard to achieve can be threatened, and take steps to protect them. This includes, but should not be limited to, increasing your familiarity with the following risk management topics:

1. Good professional practices that decrease risk.

2. Disability insurance–both through your job and on the open market.

3. Life insurance.

4. Health insurance.

5. "Umbrella policy" insurance.

6. Malpractice insurance–including additional "personal protection" riders.

7. Conflict of Interest policies and exposure.

8. A "Rainy Day" or "Emergency" Fund (see above).

9. Debt, Tax, and Investment Risk (see below). and

10. Identity theft prevention and protection (doctors are *easy* targets).

5. Manage Debt

Unless you were fortunate enough to emerge from your training debt-free as the result of family funding, scholarships, service/payback agreements, or a winning lottery ticket, you will likely have some level of financial debt. The latest figures quoted are somewhere between $150,000 and $200,000 for the *average* debt of a graduating medical student. If you have chosen a residency and/or fellowship path that involves specialization, an additional five to seven years of interest accrual can drive those numbers even higher. While we are blessed currently to receive relatively good compensation for our work, physicians are still not immune from the effects of debt. We get no breaks on the compounding power of interest. Our credit scores still take a hit if we miss a payment. And, unlike many other loans, educational loans cannot be defaulted – even if you declare bankruptcy.

With the help of your financial advisor, create an aggressive plan to pay off your debt. Regardless of your religious preferences, the wisdom of Proverbs 22:7 is indisputable: "… the borrower is slave to the lender."

6. Plan for Taxes

One of the biggest shocks to most early-career doctors is the sudden jump in their tax burden. Under the current IRS structure, the average resident or fellow can expect to almost *double* his or her effective tax rate in the first full year of practice. In addition, many of the tax breaks and deductions enjoyed up to that point may no longer apply. Indeed, I had a friend (an ENT surgeon) who found out one morning that she *owed* more in taxes for her first full year as an attending physician than she *made* during her entire chief resident year. She was so shocked and overwhelmed that she had to call in sick and take the rest of the day off!

Furthermore, taxes become much more complicated after your training years. While residents and fellows can often file the simple one-page online tax forms for their state and federal returns, the "next level" involves many more layers. You could be required to make quarterly payments rather than having taxes automatically deducted from your paycheck. In private practice, a whole slew of new taxes exist, from property tax to payroll tax to self-employment tax to environmental use tax. Investment decisions can now also be big enough to impact taxes. Financial advisors and tax accountants can help you navigate this strange new landscape.

One particular move that may make sense as your practice develops is forming a Professional Corporation (PC) or a Limited Liability Corporation (LLC). This entity can provide a means of writing off certain qualified expenses, such as CME costs, travel, advertising, and other professional expenses. While the tax implications of these decisions vary by state and by your income level, they could be a great way to help save additional money and to provide some further tax benefit. I'm not advocating that you evade paying taxes, but there are legal ways to reduce your tax burden that are commonly utilized.

Talk to senior partners and colleagues, as well as to your advisory team, about tax planning and shelter strategies that are common among doctors in your area.

7. Manage Investments

Once you have laid a firm financial foundation through appropriate management of cash, risk, debt, and taxes, you are now ready to reach potentially greater heights of wealth through advanced savings and investments. Like a professional athlete, your ability to generate current income depends upon the daily application of training and skills in a very specific job that is both physically and mentally demanding. *You will not be able to practice medicine forever*—especially if you are in a surgical or procedural specialty. Eventually, you will want to be free to retire, to do something else within medicine, or to work outside of medicine altogether. That opportunity depends entirely on your ability to follow a disciplined investment strategy.

While this book does not seek to provide even a cursory education about savings and investments, the importance of a basic *principle* of investing cannot be overstated: *you probably need help*. Often the smartest doctors are mediocre investors. You would never let a stockbroker scope your knee or manage your blood pressure. Do you really want a physician managing your money – even if that physician happens to be *you*?

Seek financial advice often from multiple sources, find an investment manager that you can trust, and continually re-evaluate your situation.

SPECIAL NOTE: In my personal experience, "investment" decisions are like a gamble, betting your money on things you think are going to happen. These decisions may or may not pay off, as the future is obviously not predictable. On the other hand, "tax-planning" decisions are generally based on laws and regulations that already exist. If tax laws do change, usually there is some level of advance warning. As such, proper tax planning might be perhaps the best investment decision you can make. Maximizing tax benefit is generally predictable, whereas traditional investing is usually not.

Bottom line on taxes and investments: get help.

8. Plan to Educate Your Kids

If you are blessed with children, one of the most important gifts you can bestow upon them is the gift of an education. Many special options exist for savings and investments in the future education of your children. If you do not currently have kids, you may still be able to invest in funds, such as 529 College Savings Plans, for future children. As doctors, we understand the value of education. It is never too early to plan for the needs of the next generation of learners.

9. Plan to Support a Cause

In health care, we spend our days caring for patients. While this great responsibility and privilege obviously counts as "helping our fellow man," many of us have additional charitable or philanthropic interests. My wife and I find much more joy and reward in giving than we do in merely consuming. Sure, it is fun to buy the nice car, the huge TV, the fancy boat, or the other "whatever" item you've always wanted as a resident. In fact, I would encourage you to pick one or two fun material things (whose prices are within reason) and "reward" yourself with them. As your financial footing becomes more solid with time, however, these material things will not ultimately satisfy you. Find a cause, and maybe several, which you can be passionate about, and share the wealth you have been blessed to receive. You will not regret it.

10. Plan to Leave a Financial Legacy

While the word "legacy" connotes end-of-career financial decisions, it is never too early to start thinking about what you want your legacy to be.

Perhaps it involves freedom from financial stress for your family. Perhaps it involves support of the institutions that helped to educate and train you. Perhaps it involves a charitable cause or a religious theme. With the power of compounding interest, coupled with a long-term goal, you could be surprised by what you can achieve if you plan ahead.

BONUS: Start Now

The best surgeons will tell you that a case goes well in the OR because it went well in their mind the night before. The best internists will tell you that they get compliance on their most challenging cases of diabetes and hypertension because they follow proven protocols. In other words, good planning generates good results. It is *never* too early to begin laying out your financial plans. If you wait until you get your first paycheck to start thinking about how you will manage your money, then you have probably already made several mistakes.

Chapter 3

MAKE-OR-BREAK BASICS OF INDUSTRY AND HOSPITAL RELATIONSHIPS

As you begin your own practice, you will quickly move from being "just a resident" to a full-fledged member of your hospital's medical staff. As such, the hospital administration will view and treat you very differently. Likewise, representatives from the pharmaceutical and medical-device industries will begin to treat you differently – mostly because you now have the power of individual opinion and you are no longer beholden to do something just because your attending told you to do it. While no early-career physician will have unlimited power with hospitals or industry, the jump up from residency is almost always significant in this area. The early stages of these relationships are critical, since first impressions and "rookie mistakes" can have significant implications for future interactions.

Industry – Opportunities

1. Product Use and Evaluation

As a "new" doctor, you will now get to make decisions about the drugs, products, protocols, and equipment you use. This might range from the type of rotator cuff anchors or ACL buttons in the supply closet to the type of fluid pumps and video towers in the operating suite. It could involve decisions about formulary drugs, code protocols, or condition-specific admission flowcharts. Many hospitals, especially if you have privileges at more than one facility, will court the newer doctors as they establish habits and practice patterns. As such, you may find that you have more cooperation from your institutions and more freedom of decision in your early days than you will have later on in your career.

You will thus find yourself inundated with requests from pharmaceutical and device-industry representatives to try their products, or with requests for you to convince your hospital or surgery center to buy them. Enjoy all of the attention that comes with this situation, but understand one thing: these representatives are *not* your new best friends. You represent low-hanging fruit to them. For example, if you use 50 gastric bands from one company in your first year, this constitutes a "growth" in business of 50 bands for that company (and its representative)—*simply because you showed up in their territory.* For industry, a new doctor is a quick-and-easy opportunity to increase drug or product sales without doing nearly the same work required to convert an "established" physician or group. Moreover, you represent a potential inroad to your senior partners, with the thinking that if the "new" doctor uses a product and does well, then perhaps the "older" ones will also change their ways.

In some cases, however, industry representatives might ask you to try a new drug, product, or device because they truly want to know what you think of it. Because you are fresh out of training, you will likely have a set of views and experiences that is different from the existing physicians in your market – a fact that can be both positive and negative. Likewise, you may find that you prefer some of your new local "standards" over those used when and where you were trained. In some cases, you may not be able to use the same brands or models with which you are familiar due to pre-existing local contracts or market patterns. In short, be ready for anything, and understand the motivations of the other players in the game.

**Until you get your proverbial feet under you,
keep your industry relationships simple and limited to good,
evidence-based use of drugs and materials.**

2. Speaking Engagements

As you build your practice in the early days, you will find that you likely have more free time on your hands than you will have once you "ramp up" to a busy schedule. If so (and even if you *don't* have much free time), speaking engagements are a great way to "get your name out" in the community. This applies both to the community at large and to the smaller medical and sub-specialty communities in your practice area.

General Opportunities

You will potentially find speaking opportunities in a huge variety of places:

1. Church or civic groups often have weekly or monthly meetings, and their "program coordinator" will be more than happy to have you come and talk to the group.

2. Local schools (especially those with pre-medical clubs, groups, or classes) are good contacts – especially if your practice has a pediatric component.

3. Many community hospitals have "outreach" programs in which staff physicians will give a lecture or seminar for interested potential patients.

4. Sports teams, clubs, and organizations (such as your local Little League or Masters Swim Team) might have an interest in sports medicine topics.

5. Physical Therapy groups enjoy hearing from local physicians and surgeons.

6. Assisted Living facilities, retirement centers, and other geriatric-specific locations can be great for doctors seeking to reach an older population.

7. Referring physicians should always be a "target" group if your area of specialization involves getting patients referred from other doctors.

Remember, the topics for such engagements can be very basic, and they do not need to be delivered like a professional Grand Rounds. Most general community speaking engagements do not involve any sort of payment, but they can be a *great* source of patient recruitment and practice building.

Industry-Sponsored

Depending upon how quickly you can develop relationships with industry, or through any pre-existing relationships, you might be able to engage in an industry-sponsored speaking event. These events are more commonly related to pharmaceutical companies than to medical device companies, but almost every company has some sort of paid "speaker's bureau" at its disposal. Your role as a speaker usually begins with a contract, followed by some sort of training program, and then a formalized opportunity to give presentations. Your audience can vary from a single physician (e.g., a specialist giving a brief "lunch talk" to a family medicine doctor), to medium-size groups (e.g., a dinner meeting with 10–20 other doctors), or to a large conference. You will usually be expected to cover certain "talking points" as part of a scripted message about the product or device. These speaking relationships can provide extra income, increase networking opportunities, and build your practice, but they obviously can also create a conflict of interest and thus should be approached very carefully. Especially if you are an employed physician, you need to request your employer's permission and oversight. In any case, be sure to have professional legal help in reviewing the contract for the industry relationship.

Academic

Just because you are now finished with your training doesn't mean that your academic career has to end. If you are taking a full-time academic position, then speaking and presenting will likely be a significant part of your required job responsibilities. In a non-academic position, however, you may still find great reward from academic speaking pursuits. Many of your patients, especially the more sophisticated ones, might find your credentials more appealing when they see that you continue to have regional- or national-level involvement with teaching other doctors.

You will also enjoy the continued networking with colleagues around the country that comes with professional society involvement. This can prove important for keeping up with national trends in disease or injury management, and these contacts are very nice to have if and when you are looking for a new position of employment. While "just being a member" of professional societies is great, you will find that deeper levels of involvement will pay higher dividends. Take advantage of your existing contacts in the academic ranks (former teachers, co-residents who enter academic jobs, etc.), and pursue opportunities through them.

3. Consulting Agreements

Perhaps the most formal arrangement a new doctor can enter into with industry outside of direct full-time employment is that of a consultant. Consultants are doctors who are paid by a company to provide end-user insight about various new drugs or products, and often they can play a role in helping design and develop these products or medication protocols. Consultants can also have responsibilities for teaching laboratory sessions or delivering talks (like a speakers' bureau). Historically, however, "consultant" was sometimes simply a nominal title used to justify large payments to physicians who used a high volume of a certain company's products – a thinly veiled form of "kickbacks." Recently, however, the federal government has cracked down on these sham relationships that essentially constitute an unethical corporate payoff to doctors.

In today's world, consulting agreements must undergo intense legal review and scrutiny in order to meet very high standards. This challenging environment, however, does not preclude their existence – and many doctors find consultant relationships challenging, stimulating, and rewarding for reasons other than the financial ones. In general, an ideal consultant will have a high-volume practice for the featured product (such as a total knee surgeon who does 500+ surgeries a year, with a majority of them using a single line of implants), and/or a "niche" practice that focuses on a rare or unique condition or procedure (such as the gynecologic oncologist who specializes in recurrent cervical cancer).

Consultants are chosen for their intimate familiarity with the nuances of a drug, a device, or a condition. But these qualities of volume and hyper-specialization are not absolute requirements, and many times a company's choice of a consultant is made simply because that doctor is particularly bright or is a charismatic speaker. If you are interested in consulting opportunities, cast a "wide net" as you investigate for them, talking to your local and regional industry representatives, colleagues, mentors, and others who have experience with or exposure to consulting.

Industry–Dangers

1. Conflict of Interest

Any industry relationship has the potential to create conflicts of interest. In short, you should ask, "Why am I doing this?" Is it for money? Is it for prestige? Is it to improve patient care? Is it to improve medical or surgical skills? Is it just for fun? You could have multiple motivations, with all of these reasons at play.

Indeed, your patients probably do receive better care if you have a healthy relationship with the vendors whose products you routinely use. Familiarity with systems and their subtleties can reduce errors, improve patient safety, and reduce costs. New drugs might truly be better than older, cheaper options. Staying on top of the "latest technology" can improve outcomes. But as your relationships with industry deepen, your true motivation may not be so altruistic. While you should always ultimately listen to your conscience when evaluating these relationships, our federal government has established a framework to help you evaluate your motives.

2. Stark Laws/Anti-Kickback

The "Stark" laws are a collection of federal acts that prohibit physician self-referrals. "Stark I" was passed by Congress in 1989 as the *Ethics in Patient Referrals Act*, and it focused on clinical laboratories. Congress passed "Stark II" in 1993 as the *Omnibus Budget Reconciliation Act of 1993*. It expanded the scope of prohibitions against physician self-referrals to include any "designated health care services." Under the broader Stark II, almost everything in the health care universe falls under the scope of the law – from x-rays and physical therapy to durable medical equipment, home health services, and even medications.

The federal Anti-Kickback statute governs items and services reimbursable by any of the federal reimbursement programs (such as Medicare). It is administered by the Department of Health and Human Services, Office of the Inspector General (OIG).

1. The most important distinction of the Anti-Kickback statute is that it carries criminal penalties – that is, *you can go to jail* for violations – whereas Stark violations only carry civil monetary penalties.

2. Stark applies to physician *self-referrals*, whereas the Anti-Kickback statute applies to *all* referral sources.

Because of the complexity of many modern employment relationships, (i.e., you could be an employee of a health system, so the definition of "self" can be somewhat muddy), any referral for any service could potentially fall under one or both of these laws.

Taken together, these laws regulate almost any financial relationship involving a physician – including ones that may seem completely harmless. Interpretations and applications of these laws are in continual flux during the current age of reform, and likely you cannot stay up-to-date on them while starting a clinical practice.

Take-home point: 1) be aware of the existence of these laws, 2) understand that they almost certainly apply to any industry or hospital relationship you might have, and 3) seek professional help from an attorney or other legal- or risk-management professional in analyzing any relationship that could fall under jurisdiction of these laws. If you don't, you may find yourself in major trouble.

An example: A recent major anti-kickback violation case involved Halifax Hospital Medical Center in Florida. The hospital reached an $85 million settlement with the Federal government in the case, wherein the hospital was found to be in violation in two main areas. First, the hospital's medical oncology program involved a reimbursement system to the referring oncologists that was linked to the volume of referrals. Second, the hospital's neurosurgeons were paid at rates almost double those of the 99th percentile of their specialty – clearly above fair market value. The size of the judgment in this case, which involved only six oncologists and three neurosurgeons, illustrates how serious an impact even a handful of physicians can have if their relationship with the hospital is out of line.

3. Sunshine Act

Congress initially passed the "Sunshine Act" in 2010 as the *Physician Payment Sunshine Act*, and its final-rule provisions were implemented in February 2013 by the Centers for Medicare and Medicaid Services (CMS). Congress instituted this act in response to several egregious conflicts of interest related to high-ranking academic physicians – such as investigators who received payments or who owned stock in pharmaceutical companies that produced drugs these doctors were currently researching under NIH grants. Likewise, many high-volume private physicians were essentially "hired guns" as "consultants" for certain device manufacturers.

The Sunshine Act requires information about payments and gifts made to physicians from industry to be published in a searchable online federal database. Although a few exceptions exist (such as one-time gifts of items less than $10 in value), almost every other item of value is covered, such as dinners, trips, cash, stocks, CME expenses, entertainment expenses, and even payments to family members.

After the published information is updated at regular intervals for a three-month period, physicians can "double check" the list of payments and gifts, and then the list becomes a part of their permanent record. As an early-career doctor, you must be familiar with this regulation, and how to navigate the searchable database. You should check it *often* to be sure that all of the information in your profile is correct.

Hospital Relationships

1. Nature of the Relationship

Employee: As a resident, you probably have or had an employed relationship with a hospital and/or a university. Once you enter practice, however, that relationship has the potential to dramatically change. At one end of the spectrum is continued *employment* by a hospital, in which you have a contract with the institution to provide services. This model could result in a high initial salary, especially if the hospital really needs a doctor in your specialty. However, the hospital could one day change its mind about you; then it can treat you like any other employee, with cuts to benefits or salary and with the potential to take away your job altogether.

Medical staff member: At the other end of the spectrum is the *medical staff member* role, in which you have privileges at a hospital and must abide by its staff bylaws, but otherwise you have no direct responsibility to the institution. This relationship is historically common in most community hospitals with private-practice physicians and surgeons, but this framework has decreased in prevalence somewhat with the recent rise in hospital employment rates. As a medical staff member, the hospital might offer you nothing more than a place to work, and likewise, it has no direct influence over your day-to-day business affairs.

Independent contractor: Although less common, the *independent contractor* role does exist in some places. This relationship falls somewhere between the other two: the hospital contracts with you for your services and pays you a salary, but it does not have full control of you like it does over an employee. This relationship is seen often in "locum-tenens" arrangements, and it usually involves a third-party physician employment company. That is, the hospital has a contract with a company that then has contracts with doctors to provide services. This model is common in areas such as anesthesiology or hospital medicine.

It is critical that you understand the nature of your relationship with any hospital at which you plan to work.

2. Call Pay

Historically, physicians regarded being on call at a hospital as part of their assumed "civic duty" and also as a way to build and maintain practices. Call responsibilities for my field of orthopedics generally involved covering musculoskeletal issues for the emergency room, seeing inpatient consults in the hospital, and dealing with after-hours issues with established patients. Surgeons were not usually paid extra for their time and effort, as it was considered "part of the job." Call responsibilities for other specialties varied by specialty type, but a similar general attitude prevailed. Everyone from internists to cardiothoracic surgeons to pediatricians to gastroenterologists had a pager, and they all saw call duty as a normal part of their existence.

In some situations, this status quo has not really changed. Employed physicians may have no choice about taking call, as it could be part of their contract. Academic institutions often rely upon house officers to cover many of the burdens that come with being on call. Older physicians often view call responsibilities as a "rite of passage" for younger physicians and as something that need not be questioned or changed.

In other markets, however, call responsibilities can be amazingly complex. In my area of orthopedics, some hospitals split call between "community" and "trauma," in which the complex, high-energy injury cases get managed by a different physician than the more common, low-energy injury or non-injury cases. OB-Gyn groups may cover call only for established patients and not cover call for "unassigned" patients. Our local cardiology group splits up call between "short" and "long" options – wherein the "long" call doctor has overnight duty but the "short" call doctor works only during the day. Some hospitals do not have an emergency room, and thus they have no need for "on-call" specialists. Mid-level providers have played an increasing role in many call arrangements. Some markets – usually those in major metropolitan areas – are so saturated with physicians that hospitals actually treat call duties as a *privilege*, and they might actually charge doctors for the "opportunity" to take call. The modern reality of call, therefore, is not nearly as simple as the "old guard" might have you believe.

As a result, hospitals nowadays usually find themselves somewhat at odds with their doctors on the "call issue." At the heart of the conflict is the fact that many physicians no longer see call as "part of the job." They often do not have any financial incentive to take call, since their outpatient practices often provide more than enough revenue. In fact, many primary care physicians no longer come to the hospital at all and have even resigned their hospital privileges. Call cases generally involve higher risk and liability, and the call population tends to have higher percentages of patients with low-paying government insurance, or no insurance at all. And, as generational attitudes about work-life balance continue to change, doctors (especially younger ones) will not give up their nights and weekends without a really good reason.

Hospitals, therefore, must usually provide some sort of financial compensation to encourage doctors to take call. Your first reaction to the idea of compensation is probably one of "let's drive that price up as high as it can go!" Unfortunately, however, call pay falls under federal Anti-Kickback regulations, and thus it must meet "fair market value" standards. In other words, for example, if the "going rate" for medium-size hospitals for call pay is $1,000–$1,500 per night for call, you can potentially get in trouble if your medium-size hospital offers you $5,000 per night. You should therefore approach call pay (and other non-financial benefits of taking call) with the same scrutiny that you would treat any other contract – and pay particularly close attention to the Stark and Anti-Kickback implications of the agreement.

One particular "call pay plan" that has recently gained increasing popularity is the "deferred compensation" model. This plan involves the hospital placing funds for each night or day of call into a tax-deferred account on behalf of the physician. After a certain "vesting" period, the funds become accessible to the physician. In theory, physicians may choose not to access the funds until their overall income level decreases (such as in retirement), thereby resulting in a lower level of taxation on the funds. This model has great appeal for older physicians, but it often alienates and confuses younger doctors. Early-career physicians usually need money *now* to pay off loans and credit cards, regardless of whether income tax rates on the money is currently higher. Be sure you understand the format of your hospital's call pay plan. If the word "deferred" is used at all, you could be in for a big and unpleasant surprise when the promise of "$500 per night" in 2015 turns out instead to be "a lump sum disbursement of $40,000" paid out in 2021 or later – with no way for you to access it before that time.

Be sure you clearly and fully understand the format of your hospital's call pay plan.

3. Committees

Most hospitals have a large number of committees. These committees could be broad in scope, such as the "medical executive committee," which is usually comprised of senior physicians who help make major decisions for the hospital. Committees exist for several "big-picture" issues like risk management, credentialing, finance, and other areas. But hospital committees might also be very narrow in scope, focusing on single topics such as trauma, infection, or blood-product utilization. Your participation in a committee is a wonderful way to become more involved in the management of your hospital. Senior physicians might consider committees onerous and wasteful – especially if the doctors are not compensated for the valuable clinical time that they must sacrifice to participate in the committee. As a new physician, however, you may have more time for committee participation. Additionally, you will build important relationships and will gradually improve your ability to influence matters positively for your patients and yourself. Start with one or two areas in which you have a genuine interest, and then move up from there.

4. Physician-Hospital Alignment

The concept of "alignment" between physicians and hospitals is a popular buzzword in the age of health care reform. In spite of their often-tumultuous histories, physicians and hospitals find themselves under increasing pressures to work together towards common goals. Effective alignment, however, is more than just simple cooperation between parties. The process of achieving alignment does not have simple, universal steps. Alignment will differ based on individual situational factors and the type of specialty involved. Ultimately, however, there are principles that underlie the concept of alignment and should be a part of any physician-hospital alignment efforts. In orthopedic surgery, alignment involves the clinical, administrative, financial, and even personal aspects of a surgeon's practice. Alignment must be based upon the principles of financial interest, clinical authority, administrative participation, transparency, focus on the patient, and mutual necessity. Alignment can take on various forms as well, with popular models consisting of shared governance and co-management, gainsharing, bundled payments, accountable care organizations, and other methods. As regulatory and financial pressures continue to motivate physicians and hospitals to develop alignment relationships, new and innovative methods of alignment will also appear. Existing models will mature and evolve, with individual variability based on local factors. Certain trends, however, seem to be appearing as time progresses and alignment relationships deepen – including regional and national collaboration, population management, and changes in the legal system. (Taken from Bushnell, B.D., "Physician-Hospital Alignment in Orthopedic Surgery," *Orthopedics*, September 2015.)

At its heart, alignment involves engaging in activities that maximally benefit both you and the hospital. While you may have little direct influence over such opportunities as an early-career doctor, you should definitely seek out a practice situation that seems to value alignment as part of its culture. Also, these concepts are not just unique to my field of orthopedics, but they apply across all specialties that involve relationships with hospitals.

Tax and Contractual Implications of Industry and Hospital Relationships

Any financial relationship that you might establish with industry or with a hospital will have Stark and Anti-Kickback implications, but it will also have *taxation* implications for you, and potentially for your practice. Industry will report payments under both the Sunshine Act and also under Internal Revenue Service (IRS) rules and regulations. Commonly, the tax form 1099 is used for independent contractor-type situations, such as speaking engagements, consulting agreements, and CME-event sponsorships in industry. It may also be used for call-pay or locum tenens coverage agreements with hospitals. This form is sent to the IRS, and it reports how much you were paid for your services. When tax-filing time comes, you must report this income on your own tax return. If you do not, the discrepancy could trigger a dreaded audit, or it can result in charges of tax fraud or evasion. This predicament is bad enough if you are acting as an individual. If you are acting as a representative of your group or your practice, however, it can become exponentially more problematic.

The issue of independent income could actually be covered in your employment contract or in the by-laws of your group or hospital. In some cases, all "medical practice-related income" might be subject to the governance of your employer (as is true in my current situation). In other words, any independent income you generate through speaking, consulting, call, locum tenens, etc., may be treated no differently than patient-care revenue. Thus this independent income is subject to taxation as corporate income or to inclusion in overhead expense formulas for your hospital or group. Failure to involve or inform your employer could result in costs much higher than the actual benefits of an activity.

Bottom line: There is no such thing as "free extra money" in modern medical extra-curricular activities and relationships. As you evaluate potential engagements that arise, understand the importance of the tax and contractual issues that they create. If you have questions, ask them. Get guidance from your employer, and also from an independent counsel. These situations are *not* ones where begging forgiveness is better than asking permission. The legal and financial costs of a mistake in this area can be huge, and they probably dwarf any of the potential benefits you may find. If you have an interest in these types of relationships, do not be afraid to say "no" if a certain situation does not feel right. More opportunities will come along.

Chapter 4

TIPS FROM THE TRENCHES ON BILLING, CODING, AND PRICING

As you begin your practice, you will take on some level of financial responsibility for your clinical activities. Perhaps your training has exposed you to the world of billing, coding, and pricing. Many residents, however, have no experience with these critical tasks. Even if you are a salaried hospital employee, how you document your clinical activities will have a major impact on how much your employer receives in return for your work. If you are in a private practice situation, optimization of your documentation and coding are *utterly essential* to your financial success. Entire companies are devoted to billing and coding education, and most professional societies provide CME-credit billing and coding resources specifically aimed at the needs of their membership. This book seeks to make you familiar with the foundations of billing and coding, and hopefully you can expand your knowledge using more sophisticated sources.

1. What is Billing and Coding?

You will hear the terms "billing and coding" thrown around a lot in business and practice management seminars. At the risk of oversimplification, we will define these terms.

- *Billing*: The process of preparing and sending a request for reimbursement for professional services to the appropriate entity responsible for payment is known as *billing*. The actual request might be called a "bill" or a "claim." While it may sound simple (and in most other industries, it is), this process is labyrinthine when it comes to health care. For example, when you go to a restaurant and eat dinner, the bill clearly goes to you or someone in your party. Imagine now the complexity involved if suddenly the dinner tab went instead to an office in another state, to be paid by an independent company that intended to pay for only about 30 percent of the actual cost of dinner. In health care, a bill might have several parties responsible for it – including the actual patient, his insurance company, his secondary insurance company, his employer, and potentially his lawyer. The initial process of preparing and submitting the claim is therefore *critical*, as errors can result in delayed payment, or in no payment at all.

- *Coding*: In an attempt to make this complicated process somewhat more efficient, several *"coding"* systems have been developed. Coding systems exist for diagnoses, procedures, services, supplies, and even for "episodes of care." Codes are used to convey information through automated data and revenue management systems, but at some point a human must enter the appropriate code into the system in order for the processing to begin. Many practices therefore employ professional "coders," whose job it is to make sure that the code-entry process is performed appropriately. Training, degrees, designations, and credentials are available for coders, like we in medicine have our own residencies, fellowships, and certifications. Proper coding results in maximization of revenue and can help with data-mining activities such as quality control and research. Improper coding, on the other hand, can result in lost revenue, inaccurate data, and perhaps legal problems, as many fraud cases begin with coding issues.

The "Alphabet Soup" of Coding Systems

Many different coding systems currently exist. While the scope of this book precludes an exhaustive review of all of them, you should be familiar with the basics.

(Apologies here to you non-orthopedists – many of the examples used in this chapter are orthopedic ones. It's hard enough to keep up with our own codes, so I don't know enough about other areas to be able to provide good examples.)

ICD-9 and ICD-10
(International Classification of Diseases)

The *International Classification of Diseases* began at a conference in Paris in 1900 when medical authorities from twenty-six countries met to formalize a massive "International List of the Causes of Death." The French government hosted conferences about every ten years to update this list, and it then turned over the responsibility for this process to the World Health Organization (WHO). The International Conference for the Ninth Revision of the International Classification of Diseases met in Geneva in 1975, producing the foundation of the current ICD-9. In the United States, we have used the ICD-9-CM system for a long time, wherein the "CM" stands for "Clinical Modification." This system uses a four- to six-character alphanumeric code to describe a clinical diagnosis. (For example, "Shoulder Pain" is 719.41, "ACL Rupture" is 844.0, and "Myocardial Infarction" is 410.9.) ICD-9-CM codes have been used for billing, data management, and research purposes.

In 1992, the WHO developed the tenth revision of the International Classification of Diseases, or ICD-10. This system is already in widespread use in many countries around the world. In the United States, however, adoption of the ICD-10 has been controversial. In both 2013 and 2014, the federal government first mandated adoption of ICD-10, but then postponed it. ICD-10 hit the American medical system on October 1, 2015 – just weeks before this book was published. There is a proposed split between ICD-10-CM (clinical modification) for diagnoses and ICD-10-PCS (procedure coding system) for hospital procedures, but the ICD-10 system and its application remains in flux. With widespread use of electronic medical records (EMRs) based on ICD-9, the "upgrade" to ICD-10 represents a major logistical undertaking and a gigantic capital expense for many health care systems and providers – factors that have driven high levels of resistance to the adoption of ICD-10. It seems, however, that ICD-10 is likely here to stay as the new standard coding system in the United States, so the next few years will doubtlessly see a great deal of adjustment as providers and hospitals transition their systems and practices away from ICD-9 to the vastly more complex ICD-10.

Current Procedural Terminology (CPT)

If you are a procedure-based specialist or a surgeon, you will make the majority of your money by doing procedures or surgery. Currently, the coding for most surgical procedures is based upon the *Current Procedural Terminology (CPT)* system. This system is owned and managed by the American Medical Association (AMA), with significant influence from various specialty societies – such as the Arthroscopy Association of North America, which has helped guide CPT policy for many of the codes in my specialty. CPT codes exist to describe many procedures, such as arthroscopic-assisted ACL reconstruction (CPT 29888) and arthroscopic rotator cuff repair (CPT 29827), but several procedures lack a specific CPT code (such as arthroscopic gluteus medius tendon repair in the hip). CPT codes can be created as procedures and techniques evolve, with hip arthroscopy probably representing the biggest recent area of change in my specialty. Changes to CPT codes are made annually and generally involve only a handful of procedures. However, most CPT codes have been around for a long time with minimal changes, so you will quickly become familiar with the CPT codes for the common services you provide.

The CPT system is a registered trademark of the AMA, and it is used almost universally by the major payors across the American health care landscape – from private insurance companies to the government programs of Medicare and Medicaid. In general, most payors require CPT codes to be linked to an appropriate ICD-9 code (for example, 29888 must match 844.0). If the codes do not match, the claim will likely be rejected. Many billing and coding programs (such as the American Academy of Orthopedic Surgeons' *Code-X*) have "matching" features designed to ensure that the CPT and ICD-9 codes link appropriately. Check with your specialty society or other professional organizations to see if they may have software specific for your area of expertise.

In addition to surgical codes, CPT codes are also used for "Evaluation and Management," or "E&M" services. This includes office visits, emergency room consultations, hospital admissions, and other professional services. The "level" of E&M coding is determined by the complexity of the visit and by the corresponding documentation. Maximizing the code level of each patient visit is a learned skill – and it is an absolutely critical one if you are in a non-procedural specialty. If you make the majority of your money through evaluating and managing patients (rather than operating on them), you must understand how to maximize your profitability through accurate E&M coding. Be careful that you do not misrepresent what you actually did, as "over-coding" is fraud and can land you in jail. On the other hand, "under-coding" is also illegal. Even though it is rarely prosecuted, it will certainly hurt you financially. Many doctors will "under-code" because it feels "safer." Do not fall into this trap. Code honestly but accurately to be sure you are appropriately compensated for your hard work.

Global Period

Many CPT codes involve a "global period" – a concept that a code (and the payment given in return) should cover a pre-operative evaluation, the surgery or procedure itself, and a standard period of post-operative follow-up (usually 90 days). For a standard office visit within the global period, no additional charges can be billed for evaluation and management. In many cases, x-rays and other laboratory studies are exempt from the global period restriction, and thus they can be billable. Be sure you understand the implications of the global period for the surgeries and procedures you commonly perform. More importantly, keep the global period rules in mind when performing atypical procedures, since some surgeries have a shorter global period or none at all. Also, the "global period" usually does not apply to most E&M codes, so non-procedural physicians are less affected by this concept.

Modifiers

The CPT system has a long list of "modifier codes" that are added to the main code to account for special situations. For example, let's say that you perform an arthroscopic meniscectomy on a patient who develops shoulder impingement from using crutches two weeks after surgery. The patient returns to see you for an unscheduled visit, reporting that the knee is doing great in its early recovery, but complaining of shoulder pain. You end up injecting the shoulder after performing a history and physical examination. You should get paid for this, right? Well, not so fast. Because the patient is within the "global period" for the knee surgery, you have to "protect" the coding and billing for the work you did on the shoulder from the global-period payment restriction. A "24 modifier" must therefore be applied to the CPT code for the visit and the injection in order for you to still make a successful claim.

Familiarity with modifiers is critical. Most specialty societies can provide you with a list of commonly used modifiers and instructions on how to use them. However, specifics of how to apply modifiers in unique situations are often the subject of billing and coding classes.

Relative Value Units (RVU)

Beginning with the Omnibus Budget Reconciliation Act of 1989, the federal government began to apply a Resource-Based Relative Value Scale to all physician services. Through the Centers for Medicare and Medicaid Services (CMS), the government attempts to assign a "relative value" to everything that we do as doctors – from surgeries to clinic visits to reading an x-ray. This relative value is quantified through *Relative Value Units (RVUs)* applied to each CPT code. For each total RVU amount, there are three component parts: physician work, practice expense, and malpractice expense. These components are often called "work RVUs," "practice RVUs," and "malpractice RVUs," and together they comprise the "total RVUs." For the Medicare formula, these components represent (respectively) around 52%, 44%, and 4% of the total. CMS will also include a Geographic Practice Cost Index (GPCI) modifier as well, which accounts for differences in overhead costs and other expenses across different geographic areas. This "weighted RVU" number is then multiplied by a "conversion factor" to obtain a final price for the service.

If you want to see how some of these numbers play out, you can use the "Physician Fee Schedule Look-Up Tool" on the CMS website (http://www.cms.gov/apps/physician-fee-schedule/license-agreement.aspx).

Many private payors will "piggy-back" the RVU system in calculating payment amounts to providers. Many will use the Medicare "total RVU" number multiplied by their own "conversion factor" to obtain a final price. Some hospitals will employ physicians, with reimbursement based on "work RVU" numbers, multiplied by a conversion factor (such as $75 per work-RVU). Because RVU determinations are updated often, you should maintain a familiarity with the RVU levels of the most common procedures you perform and the services you provide.

G-Codes

CMS also has a system of "G-Codes," which cover various other professional services. This can include medications, physical therapy, occupational therapy, laboratory tests (such as drug screens), and other services. A handful of surgical procedures can also be classified as G-codes, such as G0289 for arthroscopic loose body removal from the knee. In certain situations, use of a G-code might result in better payment for certain things. You will learn more about the specifics of G-codes as you come across these situations.

DRG (Diagnosis-related Groups)

The *diagnosis-related groups (DRG)* coding system applies to hospital billing and coding. If you are not a direct hospital employee, you will not likely have much to do on a daily basis with the details of this system. The concept of a DRG is essentially that an "episode of care" for an inpatient admission should have a single cost, like a "product" in any other industry. DRG codes exist for large groupings of procedures, such as "Major Joint Replacement or Reattachment of Lower Extremity," which could also include various partial total hip or knee arthroplasty procedures. Several different DRG systems exist, with certain variations used by Medicare, and others by private insurance companies, to determine hospital payments. Common to each system is an attempted reflection of "resource intensity," or the level and cost of the resources required to provide the care for the procedure in question. Certain coding systems include a "with/without major complication" modifier to reflect the obvious increase in resources required to care for a patient with a complication (such as a heart attack after a knee replacement). Additionally, some of these systems have modifiers for patients with major comorbidities (such as diabetes or vascular disease), again reflecting the greater resource intensity required and thus the higher required price.

ASC-Approved Codes

As techniques and equipment improve and cost pressures rise, more procedures and surgeries are now done on an outpatient basis. Indeed, in my field, even total joint replacement – a surgery that once required a two-week hospital stay – is now commonly performed as a same-day surgery. From a billing and coding perspective, however, a key component in the "alphabet soup" for outpatient procedures is the CMS ASC-Approved List. This is a list of procedures (and their corresponding CPT and G-codes) that CMS has created for which it will provide reimbursement if the procedure is performed at an ambulatory surgery center (ASC). If a procedure is not on this list, and yet it is performed at an ASC, then payment will likely be denied. CMS also has an "inpatient-only" list, including surgeries after which patients must be admitted to a hospital in order for payment to be made. Private insurers also have ASC and Inpatient lists, which may or may not exactly match those created by CMS. In the current world of shoulder surgery, for example, Medicare patients undergoing total shoulder replacement generally must have surgery in a hospital, and then be admitted after surgery – whereas many private plans allow total shoulder replacement in an outpatient, ambulatory surgery center setting. These exclusive-location lists, like many other coding systems, are in constant flux.

Be sure you know which lists your procedures are on as you decide where and when to perform them.

1. Clinical Documentation–The Key to All of It

Every doctor's situation differs slightly when it comes to billing and coding. Some physicians do their own coding, down to the details of actually entering information into the billing software. Other doctors do not code for any of their work, relying instead on a billing office or professional coder to glean information from the records. Regardless of your situation, your *clinical documentation* is the ultimate key to successful billing and coding. If you employ coders, they will use your notes to create a bill. Payors will use it in approving or auditing payments. How you describe a procedure, including the use of important "buzzwords," can either make or break the acceptance of a certain code by a payor. For example, whether you call a debridement procedure "incisional" or "excisional" in your operative note, it can result in four- or five-fold higher reimbursement for the exact same surgery. (*Generally, "excisional" is the "buzzword" that results in the more appropriate higher payment – if that is indeed the procedure you performed. Obviously, do not misrepresent what you actually did.*) As you learn more about billing and coding, you will better be able to document your examination findings and procedures in ways that support your coding processes. You can choose to actually include ICD or CPT codes in your documentation, but be sure you are correct when you do this. Ultimately, the best policy is to clearly describe what you did clinically, with the highest level of detail possible.

2. Contracting and Coding by Payor

Despite all of the complexity of billing, coding, and documentation discussed above, another layer exists in the process: contracting. For each potential payor, a contract will exist between them and you (or at least between them and your group or your employer). This contract will cover the specifics of payment for services, and it might reference an appendix, price list, or other sub-document that details the exact payment expected for each and every possible CPT or DRG code. Unfortunately, there are usually differences between each contract. Certain payors may refuse to cover certain CPT codes (this is common for hip arthroscopy in my specialty). One payor may reimburse highly for the same CPT code that another payor reimburses for only marginally. Some contracts may result in you having to use distinct codes for what is otherwise the exact same procedure – with the code based on who the patient's insurance carrier is, rather than on what you actually did clinically.

While you hopefully will not have to be an expert in contracts as you start your career, you will benefit from sitting down with your business manager or other equivalent staff member to review some examples of these contracts and to learn how they influence your daily routines as well as your billing and coding procedures.

WARNING: As you begin your career, you may be tempted to discuss pricing and contracting issues with your peers, just as you discussed interesting cases during residency or fellowship. Remember, however, that discussing details of pricing (especially with peers in the same market) can be considered *collusion*, which is illegal. Chatting a little about reimbursement issues over drinks at a CME meeting is probably harmless – but you must absolutely avoid any written or electronic conversations about details of pricing, fees, rates, etc.

3. Device and Implant Pricing and Implications

If you are in a procedural specialty, you will likely use a variety of expensive pieces of equipment, and you might even place countless expensive implants into patients. As such, you play an important role as a "cost driver" for your hospital or surgery center. (*Note – a "cost driver" is a person or a thing that creates costs or expenses for a business entity, such as the costs of gas or tires for a NASCAR team.*) You may find that equipment and implant pricing is completely beyond your direct sphere of influence—a common occurrence if you are an employee of a large hospital or health system. But you can still influence prices indirectly (as discussed below). On the other hand, you could find that you have a great deal of influence over price negotiations, especially if you have any stake in a physician-owned surgery center or procedure suite.

Because of the power you hold, even in non-ownership situations, you must always make certain that your decisions cannot be implicated as "inappropriate" under Stark or Anti-Kickback laws.

There are two main ways to impact pricing of the things you use: direct and indirect.

1. *Direct impact* involves participation in contract negotiations, meetings, product analysis, research of alternatives, and many other high-level "business" activities. It is doubtful you will be completely in charge of such matters in the early stages of your career, but you should definitely seek out such opportunities for development if you can. Especially in private practice, knowledge and familiarity with these issues will be a key to your advancement in leadership roles.

2. *Indirect impact* involves "voting with your practice." That is, many times you can choose to use a clinically similar, but economically different option. For example, you might prefer to use a certain type of anchor for rotator cuff repairs or a certain type of beta-blocker for heart rate control. One company's product or drug may cost twice as much as that of

their competitor. If you "vote" for one over the other by using it more often, you are making an indirect impact on cost and pricing. Many companies offer volume discounts and other such "sales" based on product use – including discounts on capital purchases (such as video monitors, pumps, reusable instruments, etc.). Your clinical usage will obviously affect these volume numbers.

Perhaps the biggest shock that most early-career doctors experience is the astronomically high costs of commonly used clinical items.

Looking at a price list for items as simple as tape, bandages, gloves, and syringes (let alone some of the high-level orthopedic or ophthalmologic devices) will likely blow your mind. Understanding and appreciating these numbers can be the first step in helping to improve patient care and to control costs.

Chapter 5

HOW "TO BE" SUCCESSFUL IN MARKETING YOUR PRACTICE

Some early-career physicians are blessed to be able to walk into a great situation in which they can be as busy clinically as they want to be, from the very first day on the job until the day they retire. For most of us, however, this is simply not reality. A vast majority of physicians will have to engage in marketing their practice to a certain extent at some point in their career, regardless of their specialty. While not everyone is an elective cosmetic plastic surgeon—constantly engaged in high-level marketing just to keep cases coming in the door—every doctor can benefit from applying basic marketing concepts in their practice. Depending on your practice structure, you might have in-house or contracted marketing services available through your employer or group, and this can be a great advantage. But you will notice the first five points below *focus on you,* and not on others, so every doctor (even small groups and solo practitioners) can help market their practice with a few common-sense actions.

1. Be Nice

On the last day of my fellowship—just before I left to head out into the big, wide world and start "real life" in medicine—one of my mentors pulled me into his office. He said, "Brad, I am going to tell you the secret to success." I held my breath as I waited for his words of wisdom. He looked me in the eye and said, dramatically, *"Be Nice."* Then he shook my hand and said, "Good luck in your practice." That was it. Initially, I was almost angry. I thought, *"Ten years* of extra education after college, and the secret is '*be nice?'* I could have just stopped after kindergarten!"

As I have built my practice, however, I have seen the truth of that simple statement. In my professional interactions, I tend to favor sending referrals to colleagues who are, simply, *nice people.* It also helps (a lot) if they are clinically excellent as well. But I will always choose the nice doc over the unpleasant one if his or her skill is relatively equal. Specialists tend to get more referrals from their primary care network if they are extra nice – and you will notice from **Chapter 3** that there is no Stark or Anti-Kickback prohibition on kindness.

Patients are even more influenced by the perception of the "nice" physician. Multiple studies have shown that patients have a more favorable experience if their doctor looks them in the eye, sits down, listens actively to them, doesn't look at a clock during the visit, as well as countless other basic "nice" behaviors most of us learned when we were children. Even patients who have complications will stick with their physician if they believe that the doctor truly cares about them – a fact that is conveyed by words and manners of kindness and compassion.

The Golden Rule of Marketing Your Practice = Be Nice.
Kindness is the most effective and cheapest option of all.

2. Be Available

At its heart, medical marketing is the process whose end result is a patient coming to see you. As such, the process is worthless if you aren't available when someone needs you. As your practice grows, and the reality of time as a limited resource becomes ever-more apparent, protecting and maintaining your availability can become a very complex challenge. Scheduling add-on clinics and after-hours elective surgeries has become more common for me as my patient volume has grown with more years in practice. Early in your career, however, you will find easy opportunities to "scoop" patients from more-established doctors, simply because a patient can get an appointment with you sooner. Work hard at maximizing your availability through simple steps, like providing your personal cell phone or email address to referral sources. Reach out through volunteer opportunities, take extra call or extra shifts, or assist and work alongside partners (when appropriate) so that everyone knows you are "open for business." Even as you grow your practice, try to maintain a policy of *"Yes Is The Answer"* when it comes to availability.

3. Be Capable

While kindness and availability are cornerstones of marketing success, there is likewise no substitute for the power of clinical competence. The chaos of starting a practice can quickly consume you and threaten to push your continuing clinical education into the backseat. Obviously, you must maintain the basic level of clinical ability required to do your job – but you should also seek out the things within your specialty that you are *really good at doing*. Coming out of training, you may have a good idea of where your clinical talents lie, but you might also surprise yourself once you are truly out "on your own."

In my practice, for example, I found that even though my fellowship focused on arthroscopic knee and shoulder surgery, I was actually really talented at complex open shoulder surgery – so I made this area more of a focus of my practice. This decision has paid great dividends. Remember, ultimately, that your reputation for clinical skill will be decided over time, and that *no one* becomes the most successful physician in his or her market on the first day of practice. Do your level best clinically, and the rest of the "marketing equation" becomes much easier to calculate. Likewise, don't over-reach, get careless, or take on high-risk cases too soon, as poor outcomes will cause more damage to your reputation than you may be able to repair.

4. Be Different

Marketing professionals spend a great deal of time, effort, and money convincing consumers that their client's product or service is better than that of the competition. Determining which option is truly "better" or "worse" is much easier if the choices are actually *different*. In modern medicine, many forces exist which are promoting the commoditization of our services. (*Note – "commoditization" is an economic process by which special goods or services that have uniqueness and distinct individual value are reduced to "commodities," or basic goods and services that have no distinguishable features. Applied here, "commoditization" means that one doctor is really no different from another.*) Regulatory standards, government mandates, hospital rules, financial influences, and other factors all drive doctors towards a faceless, almost robotic professional existence in which little distinction exists. In spite of the conforming pressures, most physicians have several things that set them apart – both *personally and professionally.*

Identify the positive distinctions that exist in your situation, and then capitalize upon them. This could be a clinical skill (such as a surgery that no one else in your market can do), atypical office hours (such as Saturday morning clinics), or ancillary services (such as in-office MRI or laboratory services). It might be *personal traits* such as the ability to speak Spanish or an involvement in community activities. Your distinguishing feature could be geographic advantages such as multiple satellite offices or offices on a hospital campus. It may be the fact that you participate in research, teaching, or clinical trials. You may have ties with a professional or college sports team, with a special club or group, or even with a major out-of-town health network. Whatever your situation, there is usually *something* that makes you different. If you can identify no significant distinctions about your practice, get to work quickly in pursuit of creating them.

5. Be A Pen Pal

In bygone days of health care, doctors would actually send *handwritten correspondence* regarding patient care issues. Thank-you letters from specialists to referring physicians were commonplace. Doctors actually spoke to one another over the phone when making consultation requests, rather than place a computerized "consult order." Today, unfortunately, the art of communication has been lost in many areas of the health care community. Privacy concerns and volume pressures pose powerful roadblocks. Physicians lack the time to talk, or they fear regulatory consequences for sending even a simple text message. If processed through appropriate channels, typed or handwritten personal notes can be a HIPPA-compliant part of the medical record. A quick phone call, especially when placed at an appropriate time of day, is usually deeply appreciated by the recipient—no matter whether it involves an initial request for help, an update, or a final thank-you. Just be sure not to wake your best referral source up at midnight just to let them know that Mrs. Smith's labs look great! As you market your practice, you will find that you can capture many of the core principles discussed above (kindness, availability, competence, and distinction) through "extra-step" efforts to communicate with your colleagues.

6. Be Prepared With a Plan

One of the basic concepts taught in any marketing class is the importance of the *plan*. Marketing activities – from simply "being nice" to major billboard campaigns – are infinitely more effective if they are part of a cohesive and unified marketing plan. Based upon your individual needs, resources, and challenges, a marketing plan can differ significantly in complexity and expense. If you have any training or experience in marketing, you might be able to manage your own plan – especially if the situation requires only a simple one. But if you have no marketing background and/or if you face a complex situation, you should definitely seek help in developing your marketing plan. Sources of help can be senior partners, office managers, in-house marketing departments, or external marketing firms. Be sure that your source of assistance has experience in *medical* marketing – as experience only in other areas could be downright worthless. Any marketing plan should have clearly defined goals and methods, and a non-marketing individual (i.e., *you*) should be able to understandable it.

7. Be Aware of Your Allies – *and* Your Competition

In any business endeavor – whether it is family medicine, gynecologic oncology, selling bicycles, or running a pizza parlor – you will have allies, and you will have competition. Identifying these two groups could be much more challenging than it seems at first. Apparent friends might not be as benevolent in action as they are "on paper," and you could also find allies in unlikely places. Competition, likewise, could come from directions that you do not expect, and your competitors might have strengths or weaknesses that are not readily apparent.

Allies in marketing your practice can be critical, and you must quickly identify and understand them – for the primary purpose of making sure that they *remain your allies*. Hospitals, other health-care related organizations, colleagues, and community organizations can all enjoy a mutual benefit from the success of your practice. For example, most hospitals will actively initiate media releases, advertisements, and other such traditional marketing methods when you open your practice and join the staff at that hospital – even if you are not a direct employee. Why? Because more business for you equals more business for them. Other allies might not be so obvious – such as the local high school who really needs a team doctor and is more than happy to help build your sports medicine practice in exchange for your volunteer services. These types of relationships with allies usually require some homework to "discover."

Your supposed allies might not always be the true collaborators that you expect. For example, if you practice a sub-specialty such as otorhinolaryngology in a large multi-specialty group with a big primary care base, do you *know* that your primary care "partners" are truly your allies? Do they send *all* of their referrals to you, or do they send a large percentage elsewhere? You must work hard to *understand* your allies after you have identified them. What do they want from you? How can you better help *them*? What do they truly bring to the table for *you*? Are they more aligned with your competition? If so, how can you change that?

Once you have a better understanding of your allies, you can spend more time on helping the relationships deepen and mature – hopefully ensuring that your best professional allies will remain in that role for a long time. Be sure to periodically thank your allies for what they do for you – whether by simple thank-you notes or by other means. Be very careful that any words or deeds used to express appreciation cannot be construed as potential kickbacks for referrals under the Stark or Anti-Kickback statutes (see **Chapter 4**). For example, let us imagine that you throw a lavish holiday party at the country club to say "thanks" to your top ten referring physicians, complete with personally gift-wrapped expensive party favors. Such an event could easily be seen as an inappropriate financial kickback – especially if an investigator could prove that an invitation to this party hinged directly upon the number of referrals that the invitee sent to you.

Sometimes your competitors, just like your allies, are obvious. If two plastic surgery groups exist in the same market, they are almost certainly competing for business. But how far out does one draw the proverbial line in determining a geographic area to define as a "market?" Patients could be drawn to bigger cities just a little farther away, or they may even be willing to travel very long distances (even internationally) for certain elective procedures. If they are located in Minnesota, would these plastic surgery groups consider a breast reconstruction specialist in Belize City to be part of their "competition?" Perhaps not at first, but they would if they have a proper understanding of the growing popularity of medical tourism. If three orthopedic groups all practice in the same smaller city, they too are likely in competition. But what about other competitors for their musculoskeletal care business? Physical therapists, chiropractors, massage centers, and other non-orthopedic options exist as options for patients with musculoskeletal problems, and therefore could be considered "competition" for the orthopedic groups.

Primary care has perhaps the most powerful competitor of all – the Internet. Modern patients seek a great deal of health care advice from Google or WebMD; a quarter century ago, these same patients likely would have made an appointment with their family doctor to try to get the same information. Other non-traditional entities have also entered as competitors in the primary care landscape. For example, why would a patient go to their primary care physician for a flu shot when they can get one at their local drug or grocery store while doing their afternoon shopping? Indeed, competition could come from any direction – and you must think creatively in order to identify it.

After identifying your competition, you should strive to understand it. Try to identify the strengths and weaknesses of your competition, and direct your own activities accordingly. For example, if Wal-Mart touts convenience for its vaccine program, you should counter with something along the lines of "personalized care." If medical tourism programs extol the sunny beauty of the Belize beaches, counter with reminders of the strange bacteria that live there that will infect recent surgical wounds. If you can even partially determine or predict your competitors' plans and actions, you will have a major marketing advantage.

Finally, understand that allies can become competitors, and competitors can become allies. Any time that changes occurring in a market result in differences in alignment, these types of shifts can occur. For example, if your best primary-care referral group is bought by a hospital at which you have no privileges, your allies might have just become your competitors. Likewise, if Wal-Mart needs a medical director for its vaccination program in your region, you may have just found a new ally for your practice.

**Allies and competitors can change like the winds…
so keep your eye on the weather.**

8. Be Careful When Using Technology

Modern medicine has seen dramatic changes in marketing with the rise of technology. I can still remember when it was actually *illegal* to market drugs directly to patients on television or in print. Today, many television commercial breaks feature some beautiful, happy fake patient telling you to "Ask your doctor about…." And most of us seem to receive those annoying spam emails about special enhancement drugs directly obtainable cheaply from Canada. Medical marketing has seen a revolution as the forces of direct-to-consumer marketing have combined with the power of television, the Internet, and social media.

If you do choose to engage in technology-based marketing, you must be extremely cautious. Entire courses are available to train you about web-based medical marketing, the use of Facebook or Twitter to build your practice, or the relative merits of television versus billboard ads. A detailed discussion of such endeavors is far beyond the scope of this book – but you should definitely do your proverbial homework if you choose to employ technological marketing. Technology can help you immensely, but it also has the potential to hurt you. You do not want to be "trending" for the wrong reasons, such as an embarrassing video that shows up on your practice's Facebook page when you meant to post it only to your private page.

9. Be Humble and Don't Over-Sell

One of the biggest mistakes early-career physicians often make is over-selling. While you may be well trained at a top-notch residency, you probably aren't the *best* doctor in your town on the very first day you start your practice. As such, *don't claim to be.* I am always amused when I see advertisements for a physician fresh out of training that highlight the doctor's "extensive experience" with some new technique or procedure. In my mind (and in the mind of most educated patients), that doctor has very little actual experience with *anything* as an independently practicing physician. Likewise, when doctors, clinics, or hospitals claim to be the "Best in the _____ Area," there is often no objective support of that claim. If your hospital gets recognized by *U.S. News and World Report,* the Joint Commission, or some other nationally acclaimed source, then it might be appropriate to publicize it. But claiming "best-ness" with no real supporting data can backfire on you.

In particular, beware of what I call the "poser awards." (*Note – the term* *"poser" came into the popular jargon during the skateboarding craze of the* *1980s. It basically referred to someone who acted, dressed, and talked like a* *skater – but could not actually skate at all. It now fits in our lexicon as a person* *who tries way too hard to fit in, to the point of comical exaggeration.*) In the world of medical marketing, the "poser awards" are a group of essentially faux recognitions such as the "Compassionate Doctor Award," "Patient's Choice Award," or the "Top Doctor" designation. Usually, such "prizes" are "won" simply by paying a large cash fee to a random marketing company that will make an eye-catching plaque or certificate for you to display in your office. You might fool some of your patients with such poser-esque wall decor, but your colleagues and some of your better-educated patients will likely be less than impressed.

Magazine companies are also often notorious for these types of expensive poser-marketing ploys. When I travel, I like to review the "Top Doctor" awards featured in some of the in-flight magazines. While some of these physicians are truly nationally known and respected, many of the featured physicians are doctors whom I've never heard of before. They may or may not have any actual exceptional clinical skill, but they did at least have enough cash to buy the "Best Doctor" title from the magazine's advertising sales representative. The true "top doctors" that I know usually don't need such "poser awards" because their clinical reputations and results speak for themselves. So if a random congratulatory award letter suddenly appears in your mailbox or your inbox, run away from the temptation to accept your place on the poser podium.

Likewise, do not over-sell yourself by claiming to provide services that you cannot deliver. For example, if you market yourself as a "heart expert," then you absolutely must have all of the appropriate credentials, training, and experience to provide top-notch cardiac care. An interest in cardiac health with only a basic primary care training background will not suffice. Making false claims can even have legal or licensing implications. If you claim certain expertise, you must actually have it.

10. Be an Analyst

One of the most common shortcomings of marketing endeavors is a failure to evaluate results. My marketing professor at Auburn told his students that most physicians would count a marketing campaign a success, and likely pay a marketing company a great deal of money, if that campaign simply involved plastering the doctor's face on a large billboard. A few weeks later, I laughed when I saw the face of one of my former classmates (a cardiologist) on an oversized billboard next to the Interstate – and I wondered if my friend considered that campaign a success. While such ego stroking might make us feel like we accomplished something, it probably was a complete waste of time and money. Consider for a moment:

- What was our goal in the first place – to recruit patients, or to show off our good looks?

- Did the billboard actually generate any new patients or referrals?

- Did it change the perception that existing patients might have of the physician?

- Did it do a better or worse job, relatively, than the *thousands* of ads on Facebook or Google that we could have purchased for the same price?

You cannot measure results if you do not first define them. The French philosopher Voltaire once opined, "If you want to converse with me, you must first define your terms." If Voltaire were a 21st-century marketing guru, he would probably say, "If you want to succeed in marketing, you must first define your results."

What are you trying to accomplish? More patients? More *insured* patients? More of a certain *type* of patient? More referrals from a certain area or a certain group of physicians? International fame? There can be many reasons for engaging in marketing activities, and you will waste a lot of time and money if you don't even know what you are trying to accomplish. Your marketing plan should analyze the existing situation, identify allies and competitors, investigate strengths and weaknesses, and (most importantly) define the desired results in measurable terms.

Once you have defined your intended results, you must then proceed to measure them.

- *First, you must have a baseline point.* For example, if the goal of your marketing campaign is to increase the number of patients from an affluent, desirable-demographic zip code within your market, then you must first know how many patients you already have from that zip code. Then you can measure how many *more* patients you have generated through the marketing efforts. If your goal is to generate more referrals of patients with knee pain from a certain group of primary care providers, then you must know how many patients with knee pain these primary care physicians have already sent to you.

- *Second, you must define your time frame.* Most things in medical marketing are best measured either quarterly or annually— although some things could be tracked even more closely (such as weekly data for intense or seasonal campaigns, or even daily data for things such as websites).

As you measure results, you must pre-define your "success point." In other words, decide in advance your goals for your campaign. It is human nature to say, "It's a success because we tried *really hard.*" We easily lose sight of our goals in the midst of working towards them, and we often compromise to a lower level if things are not progressing as well as we had hoped. If you want to increase referrals by 50 percent, then do not accept a 10 percent increase as success. Analyze *why* the campaign did not succeed, and do not be afraid to say that something did *not* work at all. If you meet or exceed your goals, go celebrate. If you don't meet them, then you should either revise your current strategy or implement an entirely new one.

FINAL THOUGHTS

I hope you have learned through this book about the "real world" that exists outside the bubble of medical school and post-graduate training. While it can seem intimidating and confusing, this is the world in which all of us must still find a way to make a living and put to use the skills that we have spent so many years acquiring. I went into a career in medicine because my grandfather, an internist who practiced in our hometown for over fifty years, inspired me with his lifelong example of compassion and care for our community. Medicine has changed significantly since he began his career at a time when penicillin had just been discovered and when entire billing records were kept on a 3x5 note card. In years past, doctors could almost ignore the "business" side of their practices, but that era has given way to our modern age, in which medicine and business are now inextricably bound.

Some of you might find these issues to be, at best, an annoying but necessary aspect of the job. For you, this book is designed to serve as a basic reference when you are forced to step away from the clinical realm for a moment to answer the incessant call of the "real world." For others, perhaps this book has been only a starting point for a deeper interest in the business side of medicine. For you, there are much more advanced educational opportunities available – from specialized books and webinars to entire degree programs like the Auburn Physician Executive MBA. I encourage you to cultivate your curiosity into a level of expertise that will allow our generation to confront the massive challenges that now face us on the existential level in health care. We need warriors – not just in the clinical trenches, but also on the front lines and in the command centers of medical business. Whether you watch the fight or join it, may this book be as informative and enjoyable for you to read as it has been for me to write.

Additional Resources

1. Awad K. *Physician Finance: A Personal Finance Guide For Doctors*: Upper Falls Press, LLC; 2015.

2. Baum N, Henkel G. *Marketing Your Medical Practice: Ethically, Effectively, Economically (4th Edition)*. Sudbury, MA: Jones and Bartlett Publishers, LLC; 2010.

3. Buford GA, House SE. *Beauty and the Business: Practice, Profits and Productivity Performance and Profitability*. Garden City, NY: Morgan James Publishing; 2010.

4. Bushnell BD. Developing a Bundled Pricing Strategy. *AAOS Now*. 2014.

5. Bushnell BD. Bundled Payments in Orthopedic Surgery. *Orthopedics*. 2015;38(2):128-135.

6. Bushnell BD. Co-Management Arrangements in Orthopedic Surgery. *American Journal of Orthopedics*. 2015;44(6):E167-E172.

7. Bushnell BD. The evolution of DRGs. *AAOS Now*. 2103.

8. Capko J. *Secrets of the Best-Run Practices (Second Edition)*. Phoenix, MD: Greenbranch Publishing, LLC.

9. Chorney GS, Goldfarb CA. Easing the transition from residency into practice. *AAOS Now*. 2014.

10. Dahle JM. *The White Coat Investor*: The White Coat Investor, LLC; 2014.

11. Gardner S. *Smartest Doctor in the Room: How Doctors and Dentists Are Outwitting Wall Street*: Stephen Gardner; 2014.

12. Guiliana J, Ornstein H, Terry M. *31 1/2 Essentials for Running Your Medical Practice*. Phoenix, MD: Greenbranch Publishing, LLC; 2011.

13. Hacker SM. *The Medical Entrepreneur: Pearls, Pitfalls, and Practical Business Advice for Doctors (2nd Edition)*. Delray Beach, FL: Nano 2.0 Business Press; 2010.

14. Halley MD, Ferry MJ. *The Medical Practice Start-Up Guide*. Phoenix, MD: Greenbranch Publishing, LLC; 2008.

15. Harbin T. *The Business Side of Medicine: What Medical Schools Don't Teach You*. Minneapolis, MN: Mill City Press, Inc.; 2013.

16. Huss J, Coleman M. *Start Your Own Medical Practice: What They Don't Teach You In Medical School*. Naperville, IL: Sphinx Publishing; 2006.

17. Lundy DW. Choosing an Advanced Degree Program. *AAOS Now.* 2014.

18. Martin TS, Larson PD, Larson JS. *Doctor's Eyes Only: Exclusive Financial Strategies for Today's Doctors and Dentists*. Charleston, SC: Brockport and Schoolcraft; 2012.

19. Mork T. *Medical Marketing Demystified*. Newport Beach, CA: Krome Publishing; 2014.

20. Peterson RN. What do you know about the Sunshine Act? *AAOS Now.* 2013.

21. Pho K, Gay S. *Establishing, Managing, and Protecting Your Online Reputation: A Social Media Guide for Physicians and Medical Practices*. Phoenix, MD: Greenbranch Publishing, LLC; 2013.

22. Tetreault M. *The Marketing MD: What Still Works To Attract New Patients. Plus What To Do When You Run Out Of Ideas*: Elite MD Publishing; 2014.

About the Author

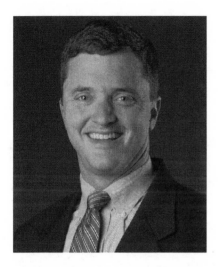

Dr. Bushnell is Vice-Chairman of Orthopaedics and Sports Medicine at the Harbin Clinic, LLC, in Rome, GA – where he specializes in shoulder and knee surgery. He also serves as Clinical Assistant Professor of Orthopedics at the Medical College of Georgia, Georgia Regents University. He holds a BA from Vanderbilt Univeristy, an MD from the Medical College of Georgia, and an MBA from Auburn University. He completed his orthopedic residency at the University of North Carolina at Chapel Hill and a fellowship in Sports Medicine at the Steadman-Hawkins Clinic in Denver. He has published over 40 articles about topics in orthopedic surgery, sports medicine, and medical business in the professional literature. He is a member of the American Academy of Orthopedic Surgeons (AAOS), the Arthroscopy Association of North America (AANA), the American Orthopedic Society for Sports Medicine (AOSSM), the American Orthopedic Association (AOA), and the Hawkins Society. He is a member of the AANA National Health Policy and Practice Management Committee. He serves as a team physician for the Rome Braves Baseball Club, Berry College, and the U.S. Ski Team. He is an Ironman Triathlete, a Little League Baseball Coach, and a Reserve Sheriff's Deputy on the Rome-Floyd County SWAT team. He lives in Rome, GA, with his wife, two children, and two Boykin spaniels. This is his first book.